How to Drive Him Crazy in Bed

Tease, Ride, and Please

By

SANDRA MISTI

How to Drive Him Crazy in Bed

Copyright © 2017

ISBN: 9781520259680

Warning and Disclaimer

Publisher Contact

Skinny Bottle Publishing

books@skinnybottle.com

Introduction

This book is based on my own little secrets on how to drive men crazy in bed. I have used every trick in this book and I am proud to say that I have succeeded multiple times.

In my attempt to be the temptress that he could never resist, I also discovered my own desires and needs. In the end, I can say that driving my man crazy in bed gave me the same satisfaction that I gave him. It made me aware of my power as a woman. It gave me the freedom to do the things that I used to only fantasize about.

You might think that satisfying a man's sexual desires is easy. After all, don't we women think that all men can think about is sex? All they ever want from us is to take us to bed and bang us. We have stereotyped men like that. Maybe there is some truth in that. However, driving a man crazy in bed is not an easy task.

It is easy to make him feel hot for you. It is easy to give him a hard-on. It is easy to actually make him cum. But to drive him crazy in bed? Nah... Definitely not easy. But it is doable.

Here is one secret to being able to succeed in driving your man crazy in bed. You have to enjoy what you're doing. You have to love every single moment of it. You have to want to keep the fire burning. You have to want him and make him want you more.

One of the common mistakes we ladies do is focusing on giving pleasure. We give everything just so he could be satisfied with the hope that we will drive him mad with wanting us. Sadly, this only works temporarily. Yes, he will want you at that moment. But will he be thinking of what happened the following day? Or even after an hour? Or once you are out of his sight? He probably will, but then again, he probably won't, right?

I have learned that fulfilling my desires is just as important as fulfilling his. Therefore I know that if he can satisfy me, I can satisfy him. I don't go for one-way traffic sexual adventures. Yes, I want to drive him crazy, but I also want him to do the same for me. I want us to go crazy wanting, loving and enjoying together.

Sex is physical. Sex is fulfilling when done right. Sex is just sex if there are no emotions involved. If no emotions are involved, craziness goes out the window. He does not go crazy. You do not go crazy. You just both got a fix, and there's nothing more to it.

Arousing him and turning him on before getting him into bed is an exciting feat. I like the idea that I can make him hard and horny even when I am just looking into his eyes. I want to see a twinkle of amusement as he realizes that I am teasing him and that I have something naughty on my mind. I love seeing that amusement turn into a desire for me, to be with me, to love me. I want to see in his eyes that he wants to tear my clothes off as much as I want to do the same to him.

Just a reminder, I am not here to give you step-by-step instructions on how you can give your man a hard-on. I am also not here to give you a list of the sex toys that you must have handy at all times. Additionally, I am not here to tell you to be a whore just so you can bring pleasure to your man. Lastly, I am not here to make you ignore your morals and do things that would make your grandmother die in shame. I am here merely to make you aware of your own powers, just as I have discovered and explored my own.

Make Him Want You First

How do you make a man want you? Well, you got to turn him on first. How? Let me count the ways.

Not all men are created equal. Therefore not all men are easy to please, and not all are unappreciative as well. Basically, you have to know your man quite well to get the feel of how he can be pleased.

Once pleased, he will want you again and again. It all has to start with the physical aspect. He already likes your looks (otherwise he wouldn't be with you). You have to make him see you in your most enchanting beauty. You have to make him feel so needy of you that he will beg you to sleep with him.

So be sexy. Men would drop anything for a sexy woman. If your man has not seen you sexy for a while, then it is probably about that time to get those revealing outfits out of the closet, or buy some if you don't have any. Dress sexy. Look sexy. Smile sexy. Laugh sexy. Talk sexy. Move sexy. Just be the sexiest you can be.

You have to make the atmosphere sexy. Create a sex-ready ambiance in the room. Make him feel like the world revolves only around that room when you are in it. Nothing else exists outside that room - just you and him and the room. You and the room - sexy, passionate, on fire and ready for the fight.

Get some wine and two glasses ready. If you want to use other stuff, then make sure that they are handy so that you don't have to get out of the bedroom or search for them in your drawers. Try to plan so you can avoid similar distractions.

Tease him. Give him hints of what you want to do to him. Make him anticipate the moment. Make him want to be alone with you.

Dress For Success

If you are planning to have a passionate night with your man, the very first thing that you need to do is to dress as sexy as you can. This does not mean dressing up like a hooker unless that is a fetish he enjoys. You can easily dress sexy and look good in bed, but turning on the sexual tension and firing up his imagination is a totally different matter.

Personally, I like dressing up. It can be really fun. But the best part is when I am taking it all off, oh so slowly. One by one, the pieces of clothing that I carefully picked up and worn, leaving my body and ending up on the floor, on the bed, on the side table, everywhere. I love watching him look at me with that intense gaze as if he cannot take his eyes off me.

Choose your dress carefully. If you intend to do a strip-tease performance you have to pick something that can be easily taken off. Very tight tops and pants might not work. They would make you act awkward trying to take them off. A short dress will do. Or a blouse and skirt - a short skirt would be perfect. Do not forget to wear a killer pair of underwear.

Set the Room on Fire

Not literally, though!

Take a good look at your bedroom. Is it ready for action? Or do you need to sexy it up a bit?

If you have a hot date that you want to end up in your bedroom, the first thing that you need to do is to make the room ready for some steamy love making. Clean up - getting rid of the clutter should be the first step. There should be nothing that says "watch your step" when he enters the room. It could ruin the mood.

I always try to create a romantic atmosphere, because I know for a fact that even I would not be aroused if the room is messy.

So set the mood by setting the room on fire. Give it a make-over, if needed. It does not have to be a renovation. New drapes, fresh bed sheets, new lighting, a new scent, some flowers, essential oils, candles, these are just some of the things that you can add to make the room ready for some action.

Do not forget to get some music ready. Nothing ignites the heat more than sensual, slow music. A good tip is to go jazzy - that always works. Go for the beat. Just try not to play real loud music.

I don't think rock music can make anyone feel in the mood for some hot passionate sex.

You may also want to get some toys ready. Whips? Handcuffs? Are you into these kinds of things? You can try them if you are up to it. This is something that you may not be ready to do. In case you are up to some kinky stuff, you may want to gather around some things that could liven up the mood. You do not have to go "50 Shades" all the way. Just have some accessories around. A glass of wine never hurts either.

Tease Him to No End

Excite him. Tease him. Tell him what you intend to do to him once you two are alone. That will surely send him to a frenzy of excitement and anticipation. He will want you right there and then. He will take you if he could. If not, he will go crazy waiting for the time when he has you all for himself.

Do the lap dance. Striptease. Set him on fire. Make him anticipate the moment until he is ready to explode. Flirt with him when you two are not together. Call him on the phone and let him know that you want him now.

You can also use SMS and email (albeit in a different way). Just give him hints that you want to do something extra nice once you get the chance to have him alone. Ask him how he's feeling and what he would like to do with you. Give him the chance to explore his own imaginations while you are out of his reach. Excite his mind as you arouse him psychologically.

You should never stop teasing in a romantic relationship. You should not stop being flirty with your lover even if you have been together for many years. Flirting on a regular basis is one of the best ways to keep the fire burning. One reminder, though, you should flirt without trying too much. It should come out naturally. If you feel like you have to force yourself to flirt or tease, you'd better stop. You won't succeed if your mind and heart are not into it. You have to be totally committed to flirting to make it work.

I can make my man go crazy just by sending him a sexy selfie on his phone. I do that before and I still do that now. I know that he likes seeing my flirty shots just as much as he likes seeing me do some naughty moves when we are together. This way I keep the fire burning.

For me, teasing should happen throughout the day and not just before sex. I can make my man stop what he's doing with just a simple peck on his cheek before I whisper is his ear just how sexy I think he is. It is this kind of small acts that drive him wild with desire for me, so when the time comes, we make love as if it were the first time we touched.

Seduce, Flirt, Explore Him and Let Him Explore You

Drive him crazy. Seduce him with your eyes, with your smile, with your words. Explore him bit by bit. Give him feather-like touches and soft kisses when you two aren't alone or in a public place.

Make him want to grab you when he cannot. Let him explore you. Let him snatch some kisses and glimpses of your skin.

Let us admit it, ladies, we all want to have that power that can drive our lovers wild, wanting and crazy in bed, right? We all want to be the temptress; the naughty girl, the fiery woman, the hungry lover.

You want to make your man go insane for you. You want him to be silly. You want him to be naughty. You want him to dream of you even when he's already with you. You simply want him to think of only you when the word sex comes to his mind. You and sex are a perfect combination for him. Sex without you is meaningless.

Light the spark. Keep it burning in flame. Never let it dim or go out. Unleash the temptress in you. Soon, your lover's eye will be fixed only upon you.

Let The Games Begin

OK, so the mood is set. You are set. The bedroom is sex-ready. You got the music and the accessories ready. Now, it is time to play. To enjoy the moment. To enjoy him. To let him enjoy you. To drive him crazy in bed. Let the games begin!

Let Your Mouth Do the Work

Sex is not something that is always planned. It can be spontaneous. Sometimes, though, when you have been doing it for a while, the sparks can fade a little. That is why it is essential to bring a little variety to your sex in order to gain the sizzle back.

One proven way to remind him that he's lucky to have you is to give him the smooches and nibbles that he fell in love with in the first place. This is also a good way of making a new man fall hard for you.

There are locking lips methods that you could try. You may like some of them and you may feel a bit awkward about the rest. The best thing is to try to experiment to know which methods work for you; for example which ones give you heat and which ones make him hold you tighter.

You must already know that the most satisfying sexual encounters begin with kisses. Locking lips with him - deep, long and lingering - will drive you both to want more. A kiss is the start of something big. It makes us aware of the needs that we didn't even know existed.

I love kissing and I love being kissed. I love the thought that when I kiss my man I can make him want me as much as I want him. When we kiss, we make the room go up in flames. We make everything and everyone else disappear - nothing matters, just the two of us. We make each other heat up in such a way that we sweat like we are already having sex. I like it when we let go and we are both gasping for breath and thinking of ways to explore each other's bodies.

Slow kiss, French kiss, almost-not-there kiss, soft pecks - there are just a lot of ways to make your kisses ignite the fire. Learn the art of kissing and get to enjoy each other.

Kissing is essential. Locking lips before, during and after making love is truly arousing, motivating and satisfying.

Learn the Art of Pre-Sex Massage

We all know about the importance of foreplay. It is the catalyst to great sex. Whenever my man complains of backaches, I am always ready to give him some good old fashion rubbing. Massaging him gives me pleasure in knowing that I can relieve him of his tiredness and I can get rid of his sores. But usually I love giving him massages because I have an ulterior motive; I want to arouse him with the soft and tender rubbing motions of my hands.

Here is how I do it. With the help of soothing music, scented oils and candles, I commence the ceremony. Once he is lying face down and naked on the bed I set to work - I rub and knead his back. Starting from the neck down to his shoulders, I slowly work my way down his back.

As I feel his muscles say bye-bye to his tensions, I start to make subtle changes in my massage actions. From semi-professional masseuse movements, I go to softer touches to act like I am finishing the session. Then I would start exploring his body. Up and down his back, making him feel more relaxed. Until he realizes that he is getting more than he bargained for. Real massage is over, erotic massage is on.

Sometimes I have to ask him to turn over. In other instances, he does that on his own. Once he is on his back, I start running my fingers through every inch of his body, focusing on the areas where he loves most to be touched - like his chest and his abdomen. My hands will linger on that spot where the tummy ends and his manhood begins. Yes, I love keeping my hands there, oily and moving sensually, as I watch him with his eyes closed savoring every touch, every caress. By that time, he will be as hard as a rock and ready for a hand-job. With the help of my hands and a few massaging tricks, I have accomplished what I want; my man is aroused and ready to take me.

Check Out The Best Bedroom Moves (Sexual Positions)

Knowing a few sexual positions won't hurt you. You do not have to be a porn star just to be able to execute these moves. It may be a good idea though to watch some X-rated videos just to see how the best moves are done.

You can also read some erotica novels if you are not comfortable watching people do it. Men are more into porn and women are more into erotica - that is a simple fact.

The 69? Why not. This position lets you enjoy him and him to enjoy you. Most people consider this position as the final act of foreplay. After touching, smooching and alternately going down on each other, going on 69 fulfills the best orals to get you both ready for penetration.

Going on top of him is probably a basic position that you have done before. Ask any guy about one of his favorite positions and he would probably say he likes his woman in the driver's seat. This position both gives you control and lets you set the pace. It gives his hands the liberty to roam and explore your body. He also gets the bonus of getting a full view of your curves. So, go on top of him and ride him like a cowgirl. Give him a show that he will never forget.

The reverse cowgirl position is something worth trying, as well. This position gives him the view he gets from a doggie, but with you in control. It may not allow a lot of eye contact or touching, but you can drive him over the edge by looking back at him once in a while as you are doing the moves.

The rear entry or more commonly known as the doggie style is one position that leaves you helpless and him in full control. The best thing about this position is that it allows him full penetrating moves. Men love this style because it makes them feel like the king of the bedroom. And let's admit it, this is the best position because we can feel their full hardness as they deeply and hungrily push with all their might. Each thrust is felt as we are wide open for him. I personally love this position as it gives my man the chance to reach around so that he can fondle my tits and play with my clit as he keeps on thrusting with high intensity. What heavenly pleasure! To be penetrated and fondled and played with. He may not see my facial expressions as he satisfies me, but I know that my moans and the way I move my ass to meet his moves truly drive him crazy. One more thing, for me the doggie style is the best way to end a round. It is rough and fast. What better way to get an orgasm than that?

Do it standing up, spoon with him or sit on him. There are ways to really liven up the act. All you need to do is to open your mind to the possibilities and trash aside your inhibitions. You are the vixen. You are the witch. You are the temptress. You are not afraid to experiment. You are up to anything that would make him mad and both of you fully satisfied.

Talk Nasty (Or Dirty, If you Prefer)

I want to say talk nasty. But basically, it's talking dirty that really turns the man on. There is something about saying dirty things during sex that really drives him nuts.

I can easily understand that not every woman feels at ease talking nasty or dirty, especially during sex. Some of us may be able to talk dirty or discuss sexually naughty stuff with our girlfriends, but we may feel a little awkward if we are to say such terms with him, in bed.

Have you tried talking dirty when your man asked you to say something dirty to him? Do you choke trying? If you don't understand the idea of talking dirty, then you may think that it is total nonsense. The truth however is that it could be the easiest thing to do. You just need to know and learn the art of dirty talking.

Eliminate the word dirty if you are really not into it. Replace it with naughty. I am not here to teach you the naughty lines to say. All I want is to make you understand that there is nothing wrong with saying naughty things to your man while having sex, or even when you aren't doing it. Say naughty things when you are sitting having dinner at a fancy restaurant and watch his eyes flash with flame. Text him with some naughty messages and wait for his equally - if not more - dirty replies.

Your subconscious could be preventing you from being totally wanton with words. But deep inside, the words are familiar to you. You say them quietly. They are present in your mind. They want to get out. Give in to the temptation of being passionately vocal. Make him feel that you can be his true bitch. Make him the happiest man alive. Say those dirty words you have been keeping up inside. Whisper. Shout. Utter the words that will make him aware that he is doing the right thing. Drive him over the edge by being the dirty talking wench that he wants you to be.

Let Your Eyes Do the Talking

Sometimes, the eyes can convey feelings more than words ever can. Send him signals through eye contact. Let him know that you want him by just giving him a sultry look, or a slight raise of an eyebrow. Give him a wink to make him understand that you are thinking naughty thoughts.

Your eyes are as powerful as your body is. One look from you should be able to make him feel the heat emanating from deep within your body. Look at him through those full lashes and he will know that you want something good - or bad - to happen soon.

Have your eyes do the roaming. Stare at him like he's the only person on earth. Strip him off his clothes with your most seductive looks. Make him feel naked. Look at him with unquenched desire in your eyes.

Eye contact is a powerful tool that you can use on him, not just to make him aware that you want him, but also to make him go crazy knowing that you do.

Go Down On Him

Men love blowjobs. Very few men would say no to a blowjob, especially when it's the woman they want that's going to do it.

One good way to drive him crazy is to start kissing him on the lips and slowly go down on his body. Featherlight caresses should accompany the kisses. Go hungry with the kisses. Then go slow. Do not be predictable. Excite him by playing with the levels of those smooches. Until you reach his manhood. By that time, it should be hard and throbbing and ready for the fight. Look at it and enjoy your accomplishment. Be proud of yourself for being able to make it stand in attention. It's saluting you, sweetheart. Give it a kiss. A very light kiss. Watch him shiver. Watch his eyes as they wait for your next move in anticipation. Then go for it. You want it, you have it, take it fully. Hear him moan. Hear him say your name. Hear him say how good you are. Yeah, he's gone crazy. Be proud.

Another way to use blowjob to drive him nuts is by doing it when he least expects it. Better yet, do it when he's not even awake to know that he should be expecting something.

Don't you just love it when you wake up and you are being romanced? I don't know about you ladies, but I surely love that. Waking up feeling your hips kissed and licked. His hands caressing and playing down there, making me moist even before I open my eyes. My body responding to his slow and careful movements, automatically. Oh, waking up to foreplay... truly heaven on earth, indeed. So, why not return the favor? Go down on him while he's still sleeping and give him something great to wake up to - a good morning blowjob. I am sure that he would not just appreciate the move, but he would also get more turned on knowing that you have once again driven him mad with the kind of sexual pleasures that you can give him.

Make Some Unexpected Moves

Play with yourself and call him when you are flushed and ready. Seeing you playing with yourself and looking so hot will surely drive him nuts. It is this kind of unexpected move that would make you look more irresistible to him.

Leave him a very naughty note telling him about a sexual fantasy that you have long been keeping to yourself. He might be surprised or he might not be. But one thing is sure, letting him know what's on your mind will make him appreciate you more. It will make him feel that he is really special. You telling him about what you desire most is going to make him want to fulfill your fantasy. The information will make him aware that he can make you feel hot for him even when he's not around.

One move that I try once in a while whenever I am in a passionate mood is joining my man in the shower. Sometimes I do it even though I know we both do not have much time before our daily routines. The thought that I only have a few minutes to make him hot is enough for me to just get in there and start giving him my 'proven-to-fire-him-up' actions. For me, some of the best quickies we had are those performed in the shower.

I also like trying some tricks in the car as we are going home. I will touch his hand to get his attention. As soon as I see the twinkle in his eyes, I know that he knows what I am thinking. I will not keep my hand on his hand. One hand would be on his hair while the other exploring down his body. I know this is risky to do on the road, but I also know when to stop. I just do this to excite him. To let him know what I want to happen once we are out of the car and inside the house.

Conclusion

Driving a man crazy in bed is an easy task if you know what to do when to do it and how to do it. There are physical and psychological aspects involved here. You can arouse him by being physically attractive - being the sexiest vixen that you can be. Or you can use some psychological tactics in making him want you more and more every day.

It is important to understand that driving him nuts for you should not be a temporary thing. It may be easy for you to get him hard and horny for the time being. But wouldn't it be better if you can drive him to the edge all the time? What if just looking at you makes him hard? What if a twinkle in your eyes gives him the signal that you want his hand all over your body? Simple things like these can heat up the moment and make him want to grab you and do you good. If you can make your man go crazy at every possible opportunity, then you have complete control over him. He is your slave even if he does not know it. You have driven him crazy with wanting you and you are still doing it to him years down the road.

I like the fact that my man thinks I am the sexiest woman alive even when we are not together. I love waking up in the morning with his emails or text messages telling me that I am the most beautiful woman in the world and that he hopes he's the first one to tell me that. That drives me crazy and I would start wishing I have him right there beside me. The best thing I could do is to just write him back and let him know how much his words affect me. How much he could make me moist and quivering with desire just by reading his messages. I would write him back about the things that I want us to do. About the things, I want to do to him. Yes, we drive each other crazy. And that is how it should be.

What we have is a passion that cannot be defined, that is limitless and that never ends. It is not just physical. It is not just about sex. It is not just craving to get fulfillment in crazy ways. It is getting satisfaction knowing that we are both hot for each other. That a simple message can take us both to the edge. That a slight touch can send goosebumps down our spines. That a light kiss can make us both wanting to tear each other's' clothes off.

You may think that driving your man crazy in bed is a simple act of being a ready and willing sexual slave. That might work, but would that make you happy? Would that fulfill your own needs? Or are you just thinking about fulfilling his needs?

What really drives men crazy in bed is knowing that they can make their women satisfied and hungry for more. We may not be aware of it, but men also do think of ways to make us happy. It could be true that they think more about sex than us. But men also have ways of making us feel wanted and desired.

As you experiment, you will learn more about your own desires and the intense ways that can make you and your man enjoy each other. You unleash the inner temptress in you. You get up close and personal with your own passionate side. This experiment allows you to have a deeper understanding of what you want in your relationship. It makes you aware that you have what it takes to be a great lover.

So experiment. Look, dress and talk sexy. Talk naughty and be a tease. Act sexy and do those hot moves. Be wanton and wild. Be his bitch and act like you have no care in the world. Be the temptress like you never imagined you could be. Do the things that you only thought of doing in your dreams. Fulfill your fantasies as you fulfill his. Tell him about the things that you want to do to him and what you want him to do to you.

Ignite the fire. Give him a hard-on and make him ready even when it is not the right moment. Give him something to think about while all he can do is to look at you hungrily. Let him know that you want his hands all over your body and you can't wait for the time when you are alone with him. Just set the mood and watch him fire up with a kind of thirst that is almost unquenchable.

Driving him crazy in bed should start before he gets you to bed. You should actually keep on it even if you are miles away from him. He should always be thinking of you in a very passionate way even at times when he should be doing something else.

Keep the fire burning by doing small sensual acts. Trying sexting him or send him steamy messages with your most recent sexy selfie. You can also try to be a bit traditional and leave him notes in strategic places like on the bathroom mirror or by attaching it to his coffee cup.

There are so many things you can do to drive him crazy. You do not have to do all of them, though. As I mentioned above, experiment and see what will work best for you and for him. Do not be afraid to try new things - keep in mind that success does not come to those who are not brave enough to try unchartered waters.

You are his woman. He has chosen to be with you. You may not think that you are the most beautiful woman in the world, but to him you're are perfect. He would not stay with you if he thought you lack what it takes to drive him nuts. You already have him. You already know that you can make him hot for you. You have already lightened up the fire. However this fire dims when there is no one to keep it burning. Take the role of re-firing up the flame when it starts to go low. You have the power to make things as hot as it was the first time you have looked into each other's' eyes. No matter how long you have been with him, you can still discover new things about each other. You can still learn more about your own desires and fantasies.

Enjoy the ride. Make the most of your adventure. Experiment. Discover. Learn. Explore. Do not be satisfied by just making him hard. Do not be content with making him cum. Go all the way and make him go insane for you.

Win a free

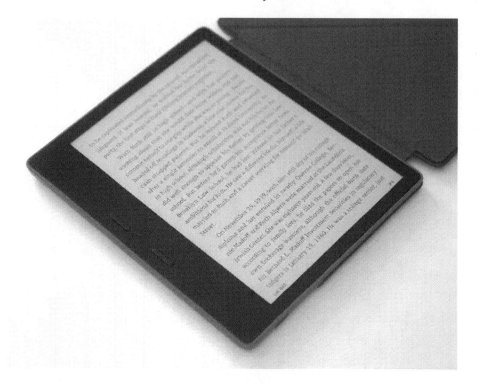

kindle
OASIS

Let us know what you thought of this book to enter the sweepstake at:

booksfor.review/drivehimcrazy

Made in the USA
Coppell, TX
30 December 2024

43717545R00018